COUGHS AND COLDS
Their Treatment by Homoeopathy

# PHYLLIS SPEIGHT

## Coughs & Wheezes
## Their Treatment by
## Homoeopathy

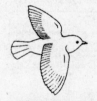

SAFFRON WALDEN
THE C. W. DANIEL COMPANY LIMITED

First published in Great Britain by
The C. W. Daniel Company Limited
1 Church Path, Saffron Walden
Essex, CB10 1JP, England

ISBN 0 85207 252 X

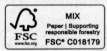
Set by MS Typesetting, Castle Camps, Cambridge

# CONTENTS

# PREFACE

After finishing my last book *Homoeopathic Remedies for Ear, Nose and Throat* I met an acquaintance who told me that her small boy didn't get many colds but they went down to his chest and took quite a while to clear up; he always had allopathic medicine and his mother was only too pleased to hear about homoeopathy.

This recalled my own childhood. I remember having pneumonia when I was about four years old, because I was fascinated by the kettle with the very long spout puffing steam in my direction, and the sheets draped around to form a little tent.

I too suffered chest colds and it was many years before I was introduced to homoeopathic treatment.

I still get the odd cold – who doesn't in this climate! – but not on my chest any more.

I always enjoyed treating children and so many of them needed remedies that would free them from chest troubles – bronchitis, asthma, chronic coughs and so on.

Here is the book to follow *Ear, Nose and Threat* and I hope the remedies will help many adults as well as children.

*Phyllis Speight*
Devon 1991

# INTRODUCTION

I have given details of forty remedies in this book as I have tried to include the most important for respiratory troubles, bronchitis and asthma.

But I must stress that the remedies given will deal with the acute conditions only.

These complaints are usually chronic – that is they return, e.g. after every cold, or in certain circumstances or weather conditions, and so on. If this does happen and the illness is not just a 'one off' then an **experienced** homoeopath should be consulted in order that 'constitutional' treatment can be prescribed. This means that the whole patient is treated, and inherited 'taints' removed in order that colds will not lead to bronchitis, and asthma attacks will not return. (This applies to all diseases, of course, and not just to chest troubles.)

As I mentioned earlier it is so important that children are given this deeper treatment to ensure that they grow up with a much cleaner bill of health. And we should not lose sight of the fact that with better health and cleaner blood-streams future generations will inherit better health.

# HOMOEOPATHIC REMEDIES

There are over 2000 fully proven remedies in our materia medica and, on thumbing through, it appears to a novice that many would help the case in hand; the physical symptoms 'seem to fit'.

But each remedy has what is called 'characteristic' symptoms which greatly help to distinguish one from another.

I have given these characteristics at the top of each remedy.

And at the end are the 'Modalities'. Modalities qualify symptoms and are very important; e.g. 'better in warm weather'; 'worse cold drinks' and so on.

In the middle I have given the physical symptoms that apply to chest and respiratory troubles which are sufficient for our needs.

This is an abbreviated materia medica which provides sufficient information for finding the remedy for acute conditions.

Each remedy follows the same format.

# POTENCY AND DOSE OF HOMOEOPATHIC REMEDIES

Homoeopathic remedies are prepared in a special way by homoeopathic pharmacists and should always be purchased from a reliable firm.

They are sensitive and should be kept in a drawer or cupboard away from sunlight and strong smelling perfumes or soaps, etc.

Pills or tablets should be handled as little as possible – usually they can be shaken into the cap of the container and popped into the mouth.

One pill or tablet is sufficient and is one dose. Put it under the tongue where it will dissolve quickly; do **not** wash it down with water and it should not be taken immediately after cleaning the teeth with a flavoured toothpaste.

In acute troubles remedies may be given frequently in the 6th or 12th potency – half-hourly if necessary for up to three doses and then less frequently, two or three hourly until symptoms improve; but the frequency of the dose depends on the severity of the condition. This dosage is only a guide and discretion should be used according to the needs of the patient. Potencies higher than the 12th should not be used by those with no experience of homoeopathy.

10

The golden rule in every case is that as soon as the patient begins to improve doses must be given less frequently and stopped altogether when symptoms disappear. This is a strict rule which must be adhered to.

If after a few hours there is no improvement then a re-assessment must be made and another search for a different remedy. This highlights the importance of study in order to find the correct remedy because it is not a good idea to change the remedy several times hoping that in the end the right one will be found. Remember, a sick person needs to be cured in the shortest possible time.

If there is no sign of improvement or the condition gets worse, then a doctor should be consulted without delay.

# HOW TO FIND THE REMEDY

Always this question is being asked and it does cause quite a problem for newcomers to homoeopathy.

However, 'The Three-legged Stool' goes some way to solving this difficulty and there is also a repertory at the end to look up symptoms and find remedies that will prove helpful.

## THE THREE-LEGGED STOOL

We have a three-legged stool in homoeopathy which helps us to prescribe, especially in acute cases. The three legs of our stool comprise well-marked symptoms in the patient and for our purpose we start with:–

### No. 1. LOCATION

Make a note of the **exact** spot that is causing problems – e.g. which side of the chest, whereabouts in the chest etc., and of course note any pain or discomfort in any other part of the area.

### No. 2. SENSATION

The second is the sensation field, the ache, pain or feeling; this should be described **in the patient's own words** (unless, of course, the patient is a baby or very small child). We should never guess because we don't know the feelings of others (even our own children) and we should not try to help by suggesting words to the one who is suffering. The sensation could be burning, pressing, itching, tight, a feeling of fullness, of fear, and so on. Add these details to your notes.

## No. 3. MODALITY

The third leg, Modality, qualifies the symptoms so that anything that makes a symptom better or worse is a modality, e.g. weather, cold, heat, eating, drinking, movement, sleep and so on.

**CAUSE** if known. This can sometimes be very useful.

*I hope the following cases will be helpful illustrations:*

A child complained of burning pains in the chest which had developed after a very bad cold. He wheezed at times and wouldn't lie down in bed at night; said he was frightened he wouldn't be able to breathe if he did.

He was restless, had a nasty cough and his symptoms got worse around midnight. *Arsenicum 6* helped this child – look it up and you will see why.

A friend complained of a cough which would not clear up. It occurred in paroxysms; the chest felt full of mucus and felt raw and sore. It was worse when she got warm in bed. A few doses of *Causticum* began the cure which took only a few days.

Look up this remedy and learn more about it.

A relative rang to say he was suffering from an attack of asthma. Said he felt very short of breath but couldn't understand why he felt 'full up' as though he would burst; he had to undo the top of his trousers for comfort.

On being questioned he said he always felt worse around teatime; couldn't bear any heat and preferred cold food. I sent him some *Lycopodium* and after a few doses he telephoned to say he was feeling better and well on the way to recovery.

Read what is said under *Lycopodium* and you will learn a little more about prescribing.

# ABBREVIATIONS

| | |
|---|---|
| ACONITUM NAPELLUS | – Acon. |
| AMBRA GRISEA | – Ambr. |
| AMMONIUM CARB. | – Amm.c. |
| AMMONIUM MURIATICUM | – Amm.m. |
| ANTIMONIUM TARTARICUM | – Ant.t. |
| ARSENICUM ALBUM | – Ars.a. |
| BARYTA CARBONICA | – Bar.c. |
| BELLADONNA | – Bell. |
| BROMIUM | – Brom. |
| BRYONIA | – Bry. |
| CALCAREA CARBONICA | – Calc.c. |
| CARBO VEGETABILIS | – Carb.v. |
| CAUSTICUM | – Caust. |
| CINA | – Cina. |
| CONIUM | – Con. |
| CUPRUM METALLICUM | – Cup. |
| DROSERA | – Dros. |
| FERRUM PHOSPHORICA | – Ferr.p. |
| HEPAR SULPHURIS | – Hep.s. |
| IODUM | – Iod. |
| IPECACUANHA | – Ipec. |
| KALI BICHROMICUM | – Kali b. |
| KALI CARBONICUM | – Kali c. |
| LOBELIA INFLATA | – Lob. |
| LYCOPODIUM | – Lyc. |
| NATRUM SULPHURICUM | – Nat.s. |
| NUX VOMICA | – Nux v. |

| | |
|---|---|
| PHOSPHORUS | – Phos |
| PULSATILLA | – Puls. |
| RHUS TOXICODENDRON | – Rhus t. |
| RUMEX CRISPUS | – Rum. |
| SAMBUCUS NIGRA | – Samb. |
| SENEGA | – Sen. |
| SEPIA | – Sep. |
| SILICA | – Sil. |
| SPONGIA TOSTA | – Spong. |
| STANNUM | – Stann. |
| STICTA PULMONARIA | – Sticta p. |
| SULPHUR | – Sul. |
| VERATRUM ALBUM | – Ver.a. |

# ACONITUM NAPELLUS

## *Characteristics*

*Fear, anxiety, physical and mental restlessness.*
*Fright – Aconite has a calming effect.*
*The sudden beginning of an acute illness with fever, anxiety, restlessness and fear.*
*Fearful for the future, of death, there are so many fears.*
*Can vomit with fear.*
*There is much tension.*
*Complaints caused by exposure to dry cold winds and weather.*

Short, dry, irritative cough during sleep.

First stages of bronchitis, cough hard, dry, painful, chest feels tight, skin hot and dry, worse at night.

Cough can be dry, short, hacking with feeling of suffocation, increasing with every respiration, with feeling of heat in lungs and tingling in chest after cough.

Dry cough brings a sensation of dryness in whole of chest; there is no expectoration except a little watery mucus with blood at times.

A dry, croupy, suffocative cough wakens patient from sleep.

Breathing becoming oppressed on least motion.

Patient is very sensitive to inspired air.

Suffocative asthma attacks occur associated with great anxiety.

Sits up, can hardly breathe, sweats with anxiety.

Anxious, short, difficult breathing.

Child may wake up in the first half of the night after exposure to cold with a violent croupy, choking cough.

A hoarse, croaking, convulsive cough is easily intensified by eating and drinking; lying down;

17

trying to talk; contact with tobacco smoke; or as the result of an emotional upset.

### Modalities
*WORSE:* Warm room; around midnight; cold, dry winds; lying on affected side; music; tobacco smoke.
*BETTER:* Open air.


# AMBRA GRISEA

### Characteristics
*Extreme nervous hypersensitiveness.*
*Weakened by age.*
*Music causes weeping.*

Hollow, spasmodic, barking cough from deep in chest. Choking when hawking up mucus.
Nervous, spasmodic cough with hoarseness and eructations on waking in morning; chest oppressed; gets out of breath when coughing.
Asthmatic breathing with eructation of gas.
Difficult breathing, shortness of breath after very little exertion, from music or from excitement. Wheezing cough.
Asthma of old people and children.
Distension with much flatulence worse after eating.

### Modalities
*WORSE:* Music; in presence of strangers (can only pass stool or urinate when alone); from anything unusual; morning; warm room.
*BETTER:* Slow motion in open air; lying on painful parts; cold drinks.


# AMMONIUM CARB.

### Characteristics
*Weak, anaemic, flabby.*
*Feeling of heaviness in all organs.*

*Weakness with no reaction.*
*Faintness.*
*Nosebleed while washing face.*

Coughs continually but raises nothing or with great difficulty.
Cough at about 3 a.m. with shortness of breath, burning in chest and palpitation.
Barking cough.
Oppression in breathing; chest feels tired; worse after any effort, ascending even a few steps, on entering a warm room.
Chest troubles of old people.

### Modalities
*WORSE:* Evenings; from 3–4 a.m.; during menses; from cold, wet weather; wet applications; washing.
*BETTER:* In dry weather; lying on painful side and on stomach.


# AMMONIUM MURIATICUM

### Characteristics
*Desire to cry but cannot.*
*Profuse glairy secretions.*

Dry, hacking, scraping cough which is worse lying on back or right side, with stitches in chest.
Asthmatic cough. Loose in afternoon with profuse expectoration and rattling of mucus. Oppression and burning in chest.
Salivation profuse when coughing.

### Modalities
*WORSE:* Head and chest symptoms in morning. Abdominal symptoms in afternoon.
*BETTER:* Open air.

# ANTIMONIUM TARTARICUM

### Characteristics

*Great weakness, lassitude.*
*Drowsiness, debility and sweat.*
*Sleepiness or sleeplessness.*
*Great accumulation of mucus in air passages with much rattling and inability to raise it.*
*Nausea, vomiting, with loss of appetite.*
*Pallor. Pale sunken face.*
*Lack of thirst.*
*Irritability.*

Every change to wet weather tends to affect larynx, trachea and lungs. There is a great accumulation of mucus, the bronchial tubes feel overloaded, consequently respiration is noisy with rattling and bubbling.

Rattling cough is weak and very little mucus is expectorated. Cough is set off by eating, with pain in chest and larynx (especially in children) and by anger or annoyance.

This remedy may be indicated in whooping cough. It should also be considered when children no sooner get over one chesty cold than another starts with rattling respiration, accompanied by weakness and debility.

Old people benefit from Antimony tart. when they suffer recurring attacks of bronchitis with much thick, white mucus and shortness of breath, when the patient has to sit up and asks to be fanned.

This remedy should be remembered for asthma which is worse at 3 a.m. causing patient to sit up, with much wheezing and rattling of mucus. Often has to be supported when in sitting position.

On falling asleep severe shortness of breath brings on fresh distress.

### Modalities

*WORSE:* Evening; from lying down at night; from warmth; in damp, cold weather.

*BETTER:* Sitting erect; from bringing up wind and expectoration.


# ARSENICUM ALBUM

### Characteristics

*Great prostration yet marked restlessness from anxiety and fear.*

*Moves from one bed to another or moves around the bed.*

*Fear – fright – worry.*

*Burning pains better by heat but patient always wants head kept cool.*

*Discharges burn.*

*Great thirst for small quantities at frequent intervals.*

*Fastidious, hates disorder.*

Catarrh travels down from nose to larynx with hoarseness; down trachea with burning and smarting which is worse coughing; then chest becomes constricted with asthmatic shortness of breath, and dry, hacking cough.

Patient is unable to lie down as he fears suffocation; better bending forward.

In asthma attacks *Arsenicum Alb.*, may help considerably if they occur soon after midnight and patient has to sit bolt upright in bed or often get out of bed for relief from walking about the room.

There is burning and sometimes stabbing pains in chest; or darting pains through lungs.

Wheezing respiration.

Asthma type cough worse after midnight, expectoration white and frothy, usually scanty.

There is great prostration and debility.

21

### Modalities
*WORSE:* At night; after midnight; 1 to 3 a.m.; cold air; wet weather; cold drinks; cold applications.
*BETTER:* Warmth, except head; loves and craves heat.


# BARYTA CARBONICA

### Characteristics
*Memory deficient; forgets in the middle of a speech.*
*Great mental and bodily weakness.*
*Childishness in old people.*
*Sadness – dejection of spirits.*
*Timid; bashful; cowardly.*
*Dread of strangers.*
*Irresolute, constantly changing his mind.*
*Chilly people, need much clothing.*
*All symptoms are worse after eating.*

Dry, suffocative cough especially in old people. Chest full of mucus but patient is lacking in strength to expectorate. Stitches in chest, worse inspiration. Lungs feel full of smoke.
Asthmatic cough.
Helps old people who take cold easily, which travels down to chest.
Cough is worse with every change in weather.

### Modalities
*WORSE:* While thinking of symptoms; from washing; lying on painful side.
*BETTER:* Walking in open air.


# BELLADONNA

### Characteristics
*This remedy stands for HEAT, REDNESS, THROBBING and BURNING.*
*Attacks are violent and sudden.*

*Many acute local inflammations; fevers with hot, burning, dry skin, so hot that heat can be felt by the hand before it reaches the skin.*

*Very red, flushed face, dilated pupils of the eyes.*

*Sudden rise in temperature.*

*Restless sleep from excited mental states which can go on to delirium.*

*There is often an acuteness of all senses.*

*Can get very angry.*

Bronchitis with paroxysms of dry, hard cough. Dry spasmodic barking cough tends to be worse at night on lying down, taking a deep breath, also worse by talking or crying and in a dusty atmosphere.

A violent tickle in larynx can cause a bout of coughing lasting minutes; feels as if head would burst.

Coughing attacks may end in sneezing.

Cough with pain in left hip.

Whooping cough with pain in stomach before attack; expectoration of blood.

Stitches in chest when coughing.

Barking cough.

The Belladonna cough is peculiar. As soon as its great violence and effort have raised a little mucus he gets peace and stops coughing. Then air passages grow drier and drier and begin to tickle and on comes another spasm as if all the air passages were taking part in it with the whoop, the gagging and vomiting.

A great whooping cough remedy with spasms in larynx causing whoop and difficult breathing.

### Modalities

*WORSE:* Touch; jar; noise; draught; after noon; lying down.

*BETTER:* Semi-erect.

23

# BROMIUM

### Characteristics
*Delusion that someone is looking over shoulder.*

Dry cough with hoarseness and burning pain behind breastbone. Spasmodic cough with rattling of mucus in larynx.
Every inspiration provokes cough.
Difficult and painful breathing. Chest pains travel upwards; cramping pains in chest. Cold sensation when breathing in.
Useful remedy in both whooping cough and croup when symptoms agree.
Asthma of sailors as soon as they come ashore. This remedy has also helped fair and fat children suffering from asthma when Pulsatilla fails.
Cannot breathe deeply enough; difficulty in getting air into lungs; gasping, wheezing, rattling. Patient must sit up in bed, feels chest is constricted.
Air passages feel as if full of smoke.
Peculiar symptom: Larynx feels cold.

### Modalities
*WORSE:* From evening until midnight; when sitting in warm room; warm, damp weather; when lying on left side.
*BETTER:* Any motion; exercise; at sea.

# BRYONIA

### Characteristics
*Complaints develop slowly.*
*Patient very irritable, do not cross a Bryonia patient, it makes him worse.*
*Pains are stabbing, stitching, worse for motion.*
*Great thirst for copious draughts at long intervals.*
*Dryness of mucous membranes from lips to rectum.*
*Faintness when sitting up in bed.*

Cold travels downwards and may lead to dry, hacking cough with much gagging and vomiting, worse on entering a warm room. Cough dry at night, must sit up, patient often holds chest with one hand and head with another.

Stitches felt in chest on breathing and whilst coughing. Cough shakes whole body and sometimes compels sufferers to spring out of bed.

Cough worse after eating or drinking; laughing, talking, smoking; on entering a warm room, and at night; any motion brings on coughing.

Sputum is rust coloured.

There may be a sensation of pressure on chest with difficulty in breathing and a frequent desire to take a long breath to expand lungs. Wants to sigh, to breathe deeply which hurts.

Difficult, quick respiration, worse every movement, caused by stitching pain in chest.

Cough with headache and feeling as if head would fly to pieces.

### Modalities

*WORSE:* Slightest motion of any kind. In a damp climate Bryonia is one of the most frequently used remedies.

*BETTER:* Lying on painful side; pressure; rest; cold things.

# CALCAREA CARBONICA

### Characteristics

*Fat, flabby, fair, faint, fearful.*

*There are so many fears, for the future, misfortune, health etc.*

*Hand is soft, cool and boneless, gives you the shivers to shake hands with Calcarea.*

*Everything smells sour – stool, sweat, urine. Taste is sour.*

*Glands are often enlarged.*

*Slow in movement.*

*Craves eggs and indigestible things like chalk, earth, raw potatoes.*

*Feels better when constipated.*

*Profuse cold, sour sweat about head. Sweats even in a cold room.*

*Feet feel as if wearing cold, damp stockings.*

*Great sensitivity to cold and cold damp weather; dreads open air, at the same time cannot bear the sun.*

*Breathless – walking slowly up a slight hill can bring on sweating and breathlessness.*

A persistent tickling cough is likely to be very troublesome at night, a dry cough. But during the day expectoration from coughing is thick, yellow and sour; or there may be slightly bloody mucus from sour sensation in chest.

Respiration rattling from excess of mucus. Suffocative spells; tightness, burning and soreness in chest worse going upstairs or slightest ascent, patient must sit down.

Chest is very sensitive to touch, percussion or pressure.

There is a longing for fresh air.

### Modalities

*WORSE:* On waking; morning; after midnight; bathing; working in water; full moon; new moon; mental and physical exertion; stooping; pressure of clothes; open air; cold air; cold, wet weather; letting limbs hang down.

*BETTER:* After breakfast; drawing up limbs; loosening garments; in the dark; lying on back; from rubbing; dry, warm weather.

# CARBO VEGETABILIS

## Characteristics

*Imperfect oxydation.*
*Sluggishness, fatness, laziness.*
*Patients who have never really recovered from a previous illness.*

Cough from cold travelling down to chest which results in a teasing cough with itching in larynx, spasmodic, with gagging and vomiting of mucus which is thin at first, then thick and yellowish green.

This remedy should be thought of for whooping cough when symptoms agree, especially at the beginning of an attack. Occasional spells of long coughing attacks.

Cough with burning in chest, worse evenings, in open air, after eating and talking.

Paroxysmal cough with redness of face made better by contact with cold air.

Carbo veg. has helped in many asthma cases when there is oppression of breathing and sufferer has to sit by an open window. Chest burning with wheezing and rattling of mucus.

Asthma with great flatulent distension.

Asthma in old people with blue skin. There is a feeling of great exhaustion and even collapse. These patients suffer from air hunger 'Fan me, I want air'.

Asthma is worse warm, damp weather and at night; stomach may feel bloated and symptoms improve on bringing up wind.

Helps people who have suffered from asthma ever since they had whooping cough.

## Modalities

*WORSE:* Evening; night; open air; cold; warm, damp weather; fats; coffee; wine.
*BETTER:* Eructations, from being fanned, cold.

# CAUSTICUM

## Characteristics

*Intensely sympathetic.*

*Depression, apprehension, timidity, irritability.*

*Aches and pains with soreness, rawness and burning.*

*Paralysis of single parts, e.g. face, throat, vocal chords, limbs; from exposure to cold, dry winds.*

*Skin dirty white; sallow.*

Cough with rawness and soreness of chest.

An annoying dry, hollow cough occurs from a paroxysmal tickling in throat, worse morning and when warm in bed. Urine may escape with each cough.

Cough can be hard, racking the whole chest. Chest seems full of mucus – feels as if only he could cough a little deeper he could get it up. struggles and coughs until exhausted or until he finds that a drink of cold water will relieve. Sputum slips back when attempting to expectorate and is swallowed; tastes greasy.

Chest feels unpleasantly tight with constant urge to take a deep breath for relief.

Pain in chest with palpitation. Cannot lie down at night.

Dryness – rawness – hoarseness – aphonia.

Cough with pain in hip, especially left.

Cough worse evening; warmth of bed. Better drinking cold water.

## Modalities

*WORSE:* Dry, cold winds; in fine clear weather; cold air.

*BETTER:* Damp, wet weather; warmth.

# CINA

### Characteristics

*A children's remedy.*
*Child very cross.*
*Bores at nose until it bleeds.*

Periodic coughs returning every spring and autumn.

Gagging cough in morning.

Whooping cough with violent, recurring spasms, cough ends in a spasm; it brings tears and pain in breast bone. Swallows after coughing; followed by gurgling from throat to stomach.

Child is afraid to speak or move for fear of bringing on a paroxysm of coughing; gasps anxiously for air; turns pale.

Dry, hollow, hoarse cough; fits of coughing with worm symptoms.

### Modalities

*WORSE:* Looking fixedly at an object; from worms; at night; in sun; and in summer.


# CONIUM

### Characteristics

*Dizziness, numbness, paralytic weakness, mental and physical.*
*Weakness of body and mind, trembling.*
*Sweats copiously during sleep or merely closing the eyes.*

A very persistent, hacking cough is caused by a dry spot in larynx with constant tickling, scraping and itching in throat and chest. It may be suffocating or paroxysmal and is worse in bed especially on first lying down. The sufferer has to sit up and hold chest with both hands when coughing.

Expectoration is scanty and only after a long spell of coughing.

Patient is worse lying down, talking or laughing, taking a deep breath and during pregnancy.

There is shortness of breath, especially when walking accompanied by constriction or pain in chest.

This remedy is helpful in some types of asthma and in whooping cough.

### Modalities

*WORSE:* Lying down; turning or rising in bed; before and during menses; from taking cold; bodily or mental exertion.

*BETTER:* While fasting; in the dark; from letting limbs hang down; motion and pressure.


# CUPRUM METALLICUM

### Characteristics

*Spasmodic affections, cramps especially in calves and sides.*

*Strong metallic taste in mouth.*

*When drinking fluid descends with gurgling sound.*

Cough has a gurgling sound, suffocative attacks worse around 3 a.m.; better by drinking cold water. Coughing spasms with constriction in chest.

Cuprum can help in whooping cough; spasms of coughing with vomiting and purple face. Better swallowing water.

This remedy has cured violent, sudden spasmodic attacks of asthma lasting from 1 to 3 hours when they can cease suddenly. Spasmodic asthma and violent, dry, spasmodic cough with feeling as though patient will be suffocated. The more shortness of breath the more the fists are clenched. Spasmodic asthma alternating with spasmodic vomiting.

**Modalities**
*WORSE:* Before menses; from vomiting.
*BETTER:* During perspiration; drinking cold water.


# DROSERA

### Characteristics
*Affects respiratory organs and is thought of as one of the principal remedies in whooping cough.*
*Cough with paroxysms following each other rapidly.*

Spasmodic, dry, irritating cough, the paroxysms following each other very rapidly, can scarcely breathe, chokes.
This remedy is often needed for whooping cough. Violent tickling brings on cough and wakes sufferer; cough deep, hoarse and spasmodic until he retches and vomits. Yellow expectoration and sometimes bleeding from nose and mouth when retching.
Harassing cough in children as soon as they get into bed at night but not during the day.
Oppression in chest so that breath cannot be expelled. Spasms of coughing follow one another so violently he cannot get his breath.
Cough worse at night.
Asthma when talking.

### Modalities
*WORSE:* After midnight; lying down; getting warm in bed; drinking; laughing.


# FERRUM PHOSPHORICA

### Characteristics
*For early stages of febrile conditions.*
*Nervous, sensitive, anaemic patients.*
*Flush easily.*

First stages of all inflammatory diseases, e.g. bronchitis, with very few indications. Breathing oppressed, short, panting. Expectoration clear blood.

Susceptible to chest troubles; bronchitis in young children, with short, painful, tickling cough.

Croup.

Hard, dry cough with sore chest.

Cough worse at night.

Asthma after midnight. Must sit up; better walking slowly and talking; suffocative fits with warmth of neck and trunk but limbs cold.

Oppression from orgasm of blood; expectoration of blood.

### Modalities

*WORSE:* At night and between 4 and 6 a.m.; touch; jar; motion; right side.
*BETTER:* Cold applications.


# HEPAR SULPHURIS

### Characteristics

*Hyper sensitive. Irritable. Impetuous. General sensitivity to all impressions, the slightest cause irritates.*

*Very sensitive to pain.*

*Feels as if wind is blowing on to some part.*

*Tendency to suppurations.*

*Sweats easily on slight exertion.*

A noisy cough and loses voice which is worse by slightest breath of cold air, or exposure to dry winds. Cough troublesome when walking. Dry hoarse cough excited whenever any part of the body or limbs get cold from uncovering; or from eating anything cold.

Croup with loose rattling cough worse mornings.

Bronchitis with rattling cough and tendency to

suffocative bouts when patient has to get up and bend head backwards for relief. Much mucus is raised with difficulty and efforts may cause nausea and sweating.

Anxious, wheezing, moist breathing; asthma worse in dry, cold air; better in damp weather.

Cough when any part of body or limbs are uncovered; cold air.

### Modalities

*WORSE:* Dry cold wind; cool air; slightest draught.
*BETTER:* Damp weather; warmth; wrapped up head; after eating.

## IODUM

### Characteristics

*Anxiety when quiet.*
*Great debility; the slightest effort induces perspiration.*
*Acute exacerbation of chronic inflammation.*
*Acts prominently on connective tissue.*

A dry suffocative cough which is most exhausting and often associated with gagging, retching and frontal headache.

Raw, tickling feeling provokes dry cough.

Croup in children with dark hair and eyes.

Croupy cough with difficult respiration. Wheezy; inspiration difficult.

Rapid, shallow breathing and shortness of breath occur on exertion.

Cough worse indoors; in warm wet weather and when lying on back.

### Modalities

*WORSE:* When quiet; in warm room; right side.
*BETTER:* Walking about; in open air.

# IPECACUANHA

## Characteristics

*Persistent nausea. Nausea unrelieved by vomiting.*
*Nausea and vomiting with clean tongue.*
*Haemorrhage bright red and profuse.*
*Peevish, irritable, impatient, scornful.*
*Ailments from vexation.*

Asthma; yearly attacks of difficult shortness of breath.

Violent asthma with panting and wheezing with great anxiety.

Suffocative cough, child goes blue in the face.

A dry teasing cough results from a very persistent tickle in larynx or in air passages. Sudden suffocative, spasmodic cough, associated with severe shortness of breath, with much wheezing and rattling in chest, accompanied by gagging and vomiting. Chest feels very tight and patient has to sit up in order to breathe.

Adults may have moist asthma and stand for long spells by an open window to get fresh air.

Asthmatic bronchitis especially in old people, and in damp or sudden change in weather. Cough with suffocation, and gagging, spits up a little blood. Has to sit up at night to breathe.

Loss of breath with cough and inclination to vomit, with nausea. Has intense nausea unrelieved by vomiting, with clean tongue.

Very useful in whooping cough if there is nose-bleed, gagging, vomiting and lack of thirst. Especially 'the infants friend' commonly indicated in the bronchitis of infancy. Child coughs, gags, suffocates, loud coarse rattling, spasmodic cough with nausea and vomiting.

## Modalities

*WORSE:* Periodically; moist warm wind; lying down.

*BETTER:* Open air.


# KALI BICHROMICUM

### Characteristics

*Discharge of tough, stringy, adherent mucus or jelly-like mucus.*
*Pain comes in small spots.*

The characteristic 'long stringy mucus' often points to this remedy.
Cough metallic, hacking, with profuse yellow expectoration, very glutinous and sticky, coming out in long strings; very tenacious masses.
Cough with pain in sternum extending to shoulders; worse when undressing.
There may be membranous shreds with cough.
True membranous croup.

### Modalities

*WORSE:* Morning; hot weather; undressing.
*BETTER:* From heat.


# KALI CARBONICUM

### Characteristics

*Very irritable.*
*Anxiety felt in the stomach.*
*Fearful. Hates to be touched; and being alone.*
*Hypersensitive to pain, noise and touch.*
*All pains are sharp, cutting.*
*Stitches may be felt in any part of the body.*
*Intolerance of cold weather.*

Asthmatic cough worse 2 to 3 a.m. or 2 to 4 a.m. Sufferer has to sit up, lean forward with head on knees for relief. Wheezing.
Cough hard and dry with stitching pains in chest. Much hawking from post nasal discharge. Lower air passages are liable to become involved resulting in

a dry, racking cough 3 to 5 a.m. and associated with bag-like swelling of the upper eyelid, more marked when coughing.

Chest feels cold. Sensation of no air in chest. Cough may be paroxysmal with much sneezing, gagging and vomiting.

Expectoration scanty and tenacious, often of small round lumps of blood streaked mucus; or of pus; increasing in morning and after eating.

Cough better sitting upright, or sitting forward, head on table or knees; rocking. Worse lying down (which is impossible); drinking; motion; draughts.

### Modalities
*WORSE:* From soup and coffee; at 3 a.m.; lying on left and painful side.

*BETTER:* In warm, moist weather; moving about.

# LOBELIA INFLATA

### Characteristics
*Nausea, vomiting and dyspepsia.*
*Symptoms from suppressed discharges.*

Extremely difficult breathing from constriction of chest.

Nausea, vomiting and shortness of breath are the general pointers in asthma and gastric affections.

Asthma with sensation of lump above breastbone. Attacks with weakness felt in pit of stomach and preceded by prickling all over.

Worse from shortest exposure to cold during paroxysm. Deep breathing relieves pressure in epigastrium.

Urine deep red with much red sediment.

### Modalities
*WORSE:* Tobacco; slightest motion; cold, especially cold washing.

*BETTER:* Towards evening and from warmth.

# LYCOPODIUM

## Characteristics

*Intellectually keen but physically weak.*

*Upper part of body thin, lower part dropsical.*

*Very apprehensive – anticipation – before delivering an address, lecture etc., but fine as soon as she gets going.*

*Likes to be alone but somebody in the next room or other part of the house.*

*Weeps when thanked.*

*Good appetite but a few mouthfuls fill up and she feels bloated.*

*Excessive accumulation of wind in lower abdomen.*

*Fullness; flatulence, distension.*

*Intolerance of tight clothing.*

*Symptoms begin on right side and often move to the left.*

*Red sand in urine.*

*Craves sweets.*

*Worse 4 to 8 p.m. (no other remedy has this as such an outstanding symptom).*

A sudden, violent, tickling cough as from a crumb or feather in larynx; cough which causes severe headaches. Feeling of constriction in chest.

Cough deep, hollow.

Cough worse going down hill; taking a deep breath and by empty swallowing. Cough at night tickling as if from Sulphur fumes.

Expectoration grey, thick, bloody, purulent, salty.

Asthma with great distension. Feels he will burst, must loosen clothes. Shortness of breath; catarrh in chest but inability to expectorate.

Severe wheezing and painting, especially walking fast or going uphill.

Stubborn bronchitis with rattling respiration with burning and soreness in sternal area.

### Modalities

*WORSE:* Right side; 4 to 8 p.m.; from heat; warm room; hot bed; warm applications, except throat and stomach which are better for warm drinks.

*BETTER:* By motion; after midnight; from warm food and drink; being cool.


# NATRUM SULPHURICUM

### Characteristics

*Feels every change from dry to wet weather.*
*Head symptoms from injuries to the head.*

A loose cough is accompanied by soreness and pain in left side of chest. Cough painful, patient may get out of bed and hold chest with both hands.

Cough worse damp weather, when lying down and at 3 to 4 a.m.

Asthmatic attacks occur with every change to wet weather, or at the seaside and are associated with bronchial catarrh.

There is often an all-gone feeling in chest and frequent desire to take a deep breath.

Asthma attacks can be violent; great shortness of breath with cough and copious, greenish, purulent expectoration; rattling in chest worse 4 to 5 a.m.

Humid asthma in adults and children. Every fresh cold brings on an asthma attack.

### Modalities

*WORSE:* Music (sadness); lying on left side; cold damp dwellings; damp weather; night air.

*BETTER:* Changing position; pressure; dry weather.

# NUX VOMICA

## Characteristics

*Very anxious, irritable, fiery temperament, impatient.*

*Can get excited, angry, spiteful and malicious.*

*Very particular and careful people.*

*Easily offended; anxious; depressed.*

*Sullen; fault-finding.*

*Over-sensitive to slightest noise; strong odours; bright light; music. Feels everything too strongly.*

*Quick in movement.*

*Very chilly and when unwell in spite of layers of clothing and hugging the fire, still feels cold.*

Asthma from every disordered stomach; connected with imperfect and slow digestion. 'Something disagrees and he sits up all night with asthma.'

Worse morning or after eating.

Colds travel downwards to chest.

Dry teasing cough with great soreness in chest.

Cough causes headache as if skull would burst.

Tight, dry, hacking cough, at times with bloody expectoration.

Spasmodic cough with retching.

Whooping cough.

Feverish when patient cannot move or uncover without feeling chilly. Cough due to tickle in larynx; worse midnight until dawn and accompanied by bursting headache; a warm drink gives some relief to cough but the act of drinking induces fresh chilliness. Shallow breathing. Cough with sensation as if something torn in chest.

## Modalities

*WORSE:* Cold; dry winds; east winds; morning; over-eating; over-drinking.

*BETTER:* Warm, wet weather; evening; after a nap.

# PHOSPHORUS

## Characteristics

*Extremely sensitive, especially to external impressions.*

*Fearful of thunderstorms; being alone; of the dark; disease; death; that something awful will happen.*

*Very affectionate; they need it and give it, yet there can be an indifference.*

*Desire to be rubbed.*

*Much weakness and trembling.*

*Burning pains.*

*Haemorrhages bright and free flowing.*

*Thirst for cold drinks which are vomited as soon as they become warm in the stomach.*

Hard, dry cough from persistent tickle felt quite low down in sternum; or in throat. Worse lying down at night if on left side.

Cough with discomfort in chest, a sense of oppression or tightness; or a weak feeling. Sometimes violent stitching pains in left side of chest.

Cough is worse from cold air, laughing, talking, strong odours, and by changing from a warm to cold atmosphere or vice versa.

May be involuntary stools when coughing. Sweetish taste while coughing.

Bronchitis with yellow blood-streaked sputum, hard, dry, tight cough which hurts chest.

Suffocative attacks occur at night.

Shortness of breath if walking against wind.

Sputum more marked in daytime; tough, yellow, rusty, purulent; sour; sweet or salty and may contain blood.

## Modalities

*WORSE:* Physical or mental exertion; twilight; warm food or drink; from getting wet in hot weather; change of weather; evening; lying on painful side.

*BETTER:* Heat (everywhere except stomach and head).

Dr Margaret Tyler says: 'Phosphorus complaints are worse from cold and cold weather, better from heat and warm applications, except for complaints of head and stomach, which are ameliorated by cold.


## PULSATILLA

### Characteristics
The temperament is mild and gentle but anger can appear, and irritability.
Tears come very easily.
Conscientious; hates to be hussled.
Loves sympathy and fuss.
Changeable in everything; in disposition (like an April shower and sunshine); pains wander from joint to joint; no two stools are alike, etch.
Pulsatilla feels the heat; they must have air; it makes them feel much better.
Cannot eat fat, rich food, it makes them feel sick.
Thirstless, even with a fever.

A dry teasing cough worse lying down; a suffocative sensation forces patient to sit up in order to get more air. Or cough may be troublesome all day and cease at night.
Cough can be loose with copious expectoration; bland, thick, bitter, greenish. Feeling of pressure and soreness in chest. Urine may be emitted with cough.
Cough caused by inspiration; or from tickling or scraping in larynx. Worse in, or coming into a warm room. There may be paroxysmal gagging and choking.
Asthma after suppression of any rash or menses; with hysteria.

41

### Modalities

*WORSE:* Warm room; warm applications. Can not bear heat in any form.

*BETTER:* Cool open air; walking slowly in open air but pains of Pulsatilla are accompanied by chilliness.


# RHUS TOXICODENDRON

### Characteristics

*Great restlessness; cannot lie or sit long in one position. Changes often for temporary relief.*
*Stiffness on beginning to move.*
*Triangular red-tip of tongue.*

Dry, teasing cough with shivering resulting from putting hands outside bedcovers, associated with a raw, scraped sensation in air passages and sometimes with taste of blood in mouth. Oppression of chest, cannot get breath, with sticking pain. Much hawking of mucus with a salty taste.
Cough during sleep.
Bronchial coughs in old people which hurt the chest and may cause a bad headache. Worse contact with cold air. Sputum may be rust coloured or small plugs of mucus.
Loose cough worse morning, tight, dry cough worse evening.
Asthma when attacks alternate with herpes labialis may need this remedy.

### Modalities

*WORSE:* Quietly sitting or lying and on beginning to move; lifting or straining; getting wet when sweating; wet, cold weather.
*BETTER:* By continued motion until tiredness sets in; warmth; dry air and weather.

# RUMEX CRISPUS

## Characteristics

*Pains coming and going, never constant.*
*Intense itching of skin, especially lower extremities, worse when exposed to cold air whilst undressing.*
*Dry, teasing cough preventing sleep.*

Dry, spasmodic cough like early stages of whooping cough.

Paroxysms preceded by tickling in throat with congestion.

Paroxysms of coughing violent on lying down, then asleep all night; cough begins again on waking and paroxysms continue through the day.

Thin, watery expectoration by the mouthful in early stages to tough, stringy tenacious mucus.

Every fit of coughing produced a few drops of urine.

Cough is worse from breathing cold air; from going from a warm room into a cold one; and at night; by pressure and from talking.

## Modalities

*WORSE:* In evening; from breathing in cold air; from uncovering.


# SAMBUCUS NIGRA

## Characteristics

*Constant fretfulness.*
*Acts especially on respiratory organs.*
*Profuse sweats accompany many ailments.*

This remedy often helps children. Child wakes, sits up, gasps for breath, turns blue; this subsides, child goes to sleep only to wake up again with another attack; this pattern continues. Child may be well when awake but sleeps into trouble. Has dry heat when asleep but profuse sweat when awake.

Sudden asthma attacks around 3 a.m.; must spring out of bed.

Chest oppressed with pressure in stomach and nausea.

Hoarseness and tenacious mucus in larynx.

Paroxysmal suffocative cough around midnight; child cries and pants for breath.

Spasmodic croup.

Sniffles of infants; loose, choking cough.

### Modalities

*WORSE:* Sleep; during rest; after eating fruit.
*BETTER:* Sitting up in bed; motion.


## SENEGA

### Characteristics

*Sensation as if eyes are too large for orbits.*
*Catarrhal symptoms of respiratory tract.*

Bursting pain in back on coughing.

Hacking cough.

Cough often ends with a sneeze.

Bronchial catarrh with sore chest; much mucus and sensation of weight in chest. Chest rattles with mucus.

There is much difficulty in raising the tough, profuse mucus, especially by old people. Chest is oppressed, worse on ascending.

This remedy helps old people with chronic emphysema, asthma and bronchitis when symptoms agree.

### Modalities

*WORSE:* Walking in open air; during rest.
*BETTER:* Sweating; bending head backwards.


## SEPIA

### Characteristics

*Great indifference to family (to husband and often children) and friends.*

*Averse to work; loses interest in what she ordinarily loves.*
*Irritable.*
*Easily offended.*
*Anxious.*
*Dreads to be alone.*
*Nervous, jumpy, hysterical.*
*Weeps when telling symptoms.*
*Depressed. Hates sympathy and weeps if it is offered.*
*Wants to get away to be quiet.*
*Weakness; weariness.*
*Pains travel upwards.*
*A 'ball' sensation in inner parts.*
*Faints when kneeling.*
*Feels the cold, must have air.*
*Gnawing hunger.*
*Craves vinegar and sour things; aversion to meat, fat, often bread and milk.*

Tendency to take cold easily.

Violent, hacking cough with retching and gagging worse on waking and also from bedtime to midnight; often desires food.

Profuse expectoration in the morning which is thick, yellow and tenacious. No expectoration in evening or there can be expectoration at night and none by day.

Oppression of chest morning and evening. Various discomforts and pains in chest are better by pressure on thorax.

Shortness of breath worse after sleep and better for rapid motion. Asthmatic cough.

Whooping cough that drags on; cough excited by tickling in larynx or chest.

### Modalities
*WORSE:* Damp; left side; after sweating; cold; cold air; east winds; sultry, moist weather.

45

*BETTER:* Exercise; pressure; warmth of bed; hot applications.


# SILICA

### *Characteristics*
*Want of grit – moral and physical.*
*Yielding, faint-hearted, anxious.*
*Very sensitive to all impressions.*
*Easily irritated over trifles; touchy and self-willed.*
*Fixed ideas.*
*Intolerance of alcohol.*
*Suppurative processes.*
*Under-nourished from imperfect assimilation.*
*Feels the cold.*

Silica is subject to colds involving air passages.
A dry cough is associated with a tiresome tickle.
Cough and sore throat with expectoration during day bloody and purulent, with stitches in chest through to back.
In chronic cases cough is violent when lying down, with thick yellow sputum which has an offensive odour.
A persistent and fatiguing cough with suffocative spasms.
Cough is better warm drinks.

### *Modalities*
*WORSE:* Morning; uncovering; damp.
*BETTER:* Warmth; wrapping up head; in the summer; in wet or humid weather.


# SPONGIA TOSTA

### *Characteristics*
*Very marked symptoms of respiratory organs.*
*Exhaustion and heaviness of body after slight exertion with orgasm of blood to chest and face.*

*Anxiety and difficult breathing.*

Great dryness of all air passages; cough dry, barking, croupy; sounds like a saw driven through a board.

Croup worse inspiring air; before midnight. Breathing short, panting, with feeling of plug in larynx. Wakes out of sleep with feeling of suffocation; loud, violent cough, anxiety and difficult breathing.

Irrepressible cough from raw, sore spot deep in chest; chest feels weak. Cough better after eating warm food or warm drinks.

Bronchial catarrh with wheezing.

Asthmatic cough worse cold air, with profuse expectoration and feeling of suffocation. Worse lying with head low and in hot room. Violent forms of asthma. Dryness of air passages; whistling; wheezing; seldom rattling. Must sit up and bend forward. Sometimes after an attack there is white, tough mucus difficult to expel. Feels as if breathing through a sponge.

### Modalities
*WORSE:* Cold dry wind.


# STANNUM

### Characteristics
*Chief action is on nervous system and respiratory organs.*
*Debility very marked.*
*Pains come and go gradually.*
*Very weak feeling in throat and chest during and after talking.*

Loose cough with heavy, green, sweetish expectoration during day.

Violent, dry cough in the evening until midnight. Mucus has to be expelled forcibly.

Cough excited by laughing, singing, talking; worse lying on right side.

Can hardly talk as chest feels sore and weak.

Respiration short, oppressive; stitches in left side when breathing and lying on same side.

Cough with influenza from noon to midnight with scanty expectoration.

### Modalities
*WORSE:* Using voice; lying on right side; warm drinks.
*BETTER:* Coughing or expectorating; hard pressure.

## STICTA PULMONARIA

### Characteristics
*Heavy pain and pressure in forehead and root of nose.*

*Excessive dryness of nose.*

Pressure in forehead and root of nose commences with every cold; this lessens or ceases when nose begins to discharge. The secretion tends to dry up quickly but there is a constant inclination to blow nose because of an irritation, without any result.

The cough is very dry, worse at night when lying down, keeping the patient awake, worse inspiration. Sticta is one of the best remedies for an obstinate cough attending, or following measles; worse towards evening and when tired. The cough is dry but may become a little loose in the morning.

### Modalities
*WORSE:* Sudden changes in temperature.

## SULPHUR

### Characteristics
*This remedy is known as the ragged philosopher.*

*Selfish, lazy and untidy people who often fling themselves into a chair with one leg draped over the arm. They are philosophical, wanting to know the 'Whys and wherefores'.*

*Skin burning with itching; worse from warmth of bed.*

*Red orifices; eyes, nose, ears, lips and anus.*

*Sinking feeling mid-morning.*

*Worse standing.*

*Discharges offensive, acrid and excoriating, making parts over which they flow red and burning.*

*Dislike of water; of washing.*

*Cat-nap sleep.*

Bronchitis with an urgent craving for air and much white frothy sputum, sometimes streaked with blood after coughing.

Cough worse at night.

Patient feels suffocated, wants doors and windows open. Difficult respiration, loose cough, worse talking and in the morning with greenish, purulent, sweetish expectoration. Mucus rattles; chest feels heavy.

Shortness of breath occurs with feeling of tightness in chest. Suffocative attacks at night with violent palpitation and great need for air.

Asthma attacks usually alternate with eruptions on the skin.

The more chronic cases with breathlessness and oppression of chest need this remedy, with a feeling of heat and rattling in chest especially around 11 a.m.; and a band sensation in chest.

Every cold ends in asthma.

Sulphur is warm, hungry, often craves fat, kicks off the bedclothes or puts feet out of bed.

### Modalities

*WORSE:* Warmth of bed; morning.

*BETTER:* Dry, warm weather.

49

# VERATRUM ALBUM

### Characteristics

*Delusions of impending misfortune.*

*Collapse; weakness, with blue skin and extreme coldness.*

*Cold sweat on forehead.*

*Profuse retching and vomiting.*

This is another remedy that is particularly helpful in elderly people with chronic bronchitis when there is much rattling in the chest and mucus in bronchial tubes.

Wheezing cough.

Cough may sound hollow from tickling low down; face becomes blue. Loud, barking stomach cough is followed by eructations of gas. Urine escapes when coughing.

Coughing starts after drinking, especially cold water.

Coughs on entering a warm room from cold air.

### Modalities

*WORSE:* At night; wet, cold weather.

*BETTER:* Warmth; walking.

# CHARACTERISTICS

AFFECTIONATE: Phos.
AGE WEAKENED BY: Ambr.
AIR, MUST HAVE: Puls.; Sep.
   " OPEN, DREADS: Calc.c.
AILMENTS FROM VEXATION: Ipec.
ALONE, HATES TO BE: Kali c.
     " LIKES TO BE, BUT SOMEBODY IN
  NEXT ROOM: Lyc.
ANTICIPATION: Lyc.
ANXIETY: Acon.; Ars.a.; Kali c.; Nux v.; Sep.;
  Sil.; Spong.
     " WHEN QUIET: Iod.
APPREHENSIVE: Caust.; Lyc.
AVERSION TO FATS: Sep.
     "   " MEAT: Sep.
BALL, SENSATION IN INNER PARTS: Sep.
BASHFUL: Bar.c.
BLOATED FROM LITTLE FOOD: Lyc.
BODY, UPPER PART THIN: Lyc.
   " LOWER PART DROPSICAL: Lyc.
BREATHING DIFFICULT: Spong.
BREATHLESS, WALKING EVEN SLOWLY UP
  HILL: Calc.c.
CAREFUL: Nux v.
CHANGEABLE IN EVERYTHING: Puls.
CHILD BORES AT NOSE: Cina.
CHILDREN'S REMEDY: Cina.

CHILDISHNESS IN OLD PEOPLE: Bar.c.
CHILLY: Bar.c.; Nux v.
COMPLAINTS DEVELOP SLOWLY: Bry.
CONSCIENTIOUS: Puls.
COWARDLY: Bar.c.
CRAVES EGGS: Calc.c.
    ″     CRAVES INDIGESTIBLE THINGS:
Calc.c.
    ″     SOUR THINGS: Sep.
    ″     SWEETS: Lyc.
    ″     VINEGAR: Sep.
CRY, DESIRES TO BUT CANNOT: Amm.m.
DEBILITY: Amm.c.; Ant.t.; Iod.; Stann.
DELIRIUM: Bell.
DELUSION THAT SOMEONE IS LOOKING
   OVER SHOULDER: Brom.
DEPRESSION: Caust.; Nux v.; Sep.
DISCHARGES ACRID: Sul.
        ″     BURNING: Ars.a.
        ″     EXCORIATING: Sul.
        ″     OFFENSIVE: Sul.
        ″     STRINGY: Kali b.
        ″     TOUGH: Kali b.
DREADS TO BE ALONE: Sep.
    ″    STRANGERS: Bar.c.
DROWSINESS: Amm.m.; Ant.t.
DRYNESS OF MUCOUS MEMBRANES: Bry.
    ″    EXCESSIVE, OF NOSE: Sticta p.
DYSPEPSIA: Lob.
EXCITED: Nux v.
EXHAUSTION: Spong.
FACE RED AND FLUSHED: Bell.
FAINT: Calc.c.
    ″    HEARTED: Sil.
    ″    WHEN KNEELING: Sep.
    ″    ON RAISING HEAD: Bry.
FAIR: Calc.c.

FASTIDIOUS: Ars.a.

FAT: Calc.; Carb.v.

FAULT-FINDING: Nux v.

FEAR OF THE DARK: Phos.

" DEATH: Acon.; Phos.

" THE FUTURE: Acon.

" THUNDER: Phos.

FEARFUL: Acon.; Ars.a.; Calc.c.; Kali c.; Phos.; Sep.

FEBRILE CONDITIONS, EARLY STAGES OF: Ferr.p.

FEET FEEL AS IF WEARING COLD, DAMP STOCKINGS: Calc.c.

FEVERS: Bell.

FIERY TEMPER: Nux v.

FLABBY: Calc.c.

FOODS, CANNOT EAT FAT: Puls.

" " " RICH: Puls.

FRETFULNESS, CONSTANT: Samb.

FRIGHT: Acon.; Ars.a.

FUSS, LOVES: Puls.

GLOOMY: Amm.c.

GRIT, WANT OF: Sil.

HAND FEELS BONELESS: Calc.c.

HAEMORRHAGE BRIGHT RED AND PRO-FUSE: Ipec.

HEAVINESS OF BODY AFTER SLIGHT EXER-TION: Spong.

" " ALL ORGANS: Amm.c.

HUNGER, GNAWING: Sep.

HYPER SENSITIVE TO NOISE: Kali c.

" " " PAIN: Kali c.

" " " TOUCH: Kali c.

HYSTERICAL: Sep.

IDEAS FIXED: Sil.

ILL-HUMOURED: Amm.c.

ILLNESS, NEVER RECOVERED FROM PRE-
  VIOUS: Carb.v.

IMPATIENT: Ipec.; Nux v.

IMPETUOUS: Hep.s.

IMPERFECT OXYDATION: Carb.v.

INDIFFERENCE: Sep.

INFLAMMATIONS: Bell.

INFLAMMATION CHRONIC, ACUTE EXACER-
  BATION OF: Iod.

INTELLECTUALLY KEEN: Lyc.

INTOLERANCE OF ALCOHOL: Sil.

       "       " TIGHT CLOTHING: Lyc.

IRRESOLUTE: Bar.c.

IRRITABILITY: Ant.t.; Bry.; Caust.; Hep.s.; Ipec.;
  Kali c.; Nux v.; Puls.; Sep.; Sil.

LASSITUDE: Ant.t.

LAZY: Carb.v.; Sul.

MALICIOUS: Nux v.

METALLIC TASTE STRONG: Cupr.

MEMORY DEFICIENT: Bar.c.

MOVEMENT SLOW: Calc.c.

MUCUS, GREAT ACCUMULATION WITH
  MUCH RATTLING: Ant.t.

MUSIC CAUSES WEEPING: Ambr.

NAUSEA: Lob.

    "    PERSISTENT: Ipec.

    "    UNRELIEVED BY VOMITING: Ipec.

    "    AND VOMITING WITH CLEAN
  TONGUE: Ipec.

NERVOUS: Ferr.p.; Sep.

    "      HYPER-SENSITIVENESS: Ambr.

    "      SYSTEM AND RESPIRATORY
  ORGANS, CHIEF ACTION ON: Stann.

NOURISHED, UNDER FROM IMPERFECT
  ASSIMILATION: Sil.

NUMBNESS: Con.

OFFENDED, EASILY: Nux v.; Sep.

ORIFICES RED: Sul.
PAINS BURNING: Caust.
     "      "    BUT BETTER HEAT: Ars.a.
   " CUTTING: Kali c.
   " HEAVY (FEELING) AT ROOT OF
NOSE: Sticta p.
   " RAW: Caust.
   " SHARP: Kali c.
   " SORE: Caust.
   " IN SMALL SPOTS: Kali b.
   " STITCHING: Bry.; Kali c.
   " TEARING: Bry.
   " COME AND GO GRADUALLY: Stann.
PALLOR: Ant.t.
PARALYSIS OF SINGLE PARTS: Caust.
PARTICULAR: Nux v.
PEEVISH: Ipec.
PHILOSOPHICAL: Sul.
PHYSICALLY WEAK: Ant.t.; Bar.c.; Lyc.
PROSTRATION: Ars.a.
QUICK IN MOVEMENT: Nux v.
RESPIRATORY ORGANS, ACTS ON: Samb.
     "      "    MARKED
  SYMPTOMS: Spong.
RESPIRATORY TRACT, CATARRHAL
  SYMPTOMS: Sen.
RESTLESSNESS: Acon.; Ars.a.; Rhus t.
     "    IN SLEEP: Bell.
RUBBED, DESIRE TO BE: Phos.
SADNESS: Bar.c.
SAND, RED IN URINE: Lyc.
SCORNFUL: Ipec.
SECRETIONS PROFUSE, GLARY: Amm.m.
SELFISH: Sul.
SELF-WILLED: Sil.
SENSATION AS IF EYES TOO LARGE FOR
  ORBITS: Sen.

SENSITIVE: Ferr.p.; Hep.s.; Nux v.; Phos.

    "       OVER, TO NOISE: Nux v.

    "       TO ALL IMPRESSIONS: Sil.

SINKING FEELING MID-MORNING: Sul.

SKIN BURNING: Bell.; Sul.

  "   DIRTY: Caust.

  "   DRY: Bell.

  "   HOT: Bell.

  "   ITCHING: Sul.

  "   SALLOW: Caust.

  "   WHITE: Caust.

SLEEP, CAT-NAP: Sul.

SLUGGISHNESS: Carb.v.

SOMNOLENCE: Amm.c.

SPITEFUL: Nux v.

STIFFNESS ON BEGINNING TO MOVE: Rhus t.

STOOL SOUR: Calc.c.

SUDDENNESS OF SYMPTOMS: Acon.; Bell.

SULLEN: Nux v.

SUPPURATIONS, TENDENCY TO: Hep.s.

SWEAT, COLD: Calc.c.

    "    EASILY: Hep.s.

    "    EVEN IN COLD ROOM: Calc.c.

    "    PROFUSE: Ant.t.; Calc.c.; Con.; Samb.

    "    SOUR: Calc.c.

SYMPATHY, LOATHES: Sep.

    "      LOVES: Puls.

SYMPATHETIC: Caust.

SYMPTOMS ON RIGHT SIDE: Lyc.

TASTE SOUR: Calc.c.

TEARS COME EASILY: Puls.

TEMPERATURE, SUDDEN RISE IN: Bell.

TEMPERAMENT GENTLE: Puls.

    "       MILD: Puls.

TENSION: Acon.

THIRST FOR COLD DRINKS VOMITED AS
   SOON AS IN STOMACH: Phos.
THIRST EXCESSIVE FOR LONG DRAUGHTS:
   Bry.
       "        "        "  SMALL
   QUANTITIES: Ars.a.
THIRSTLESS: Ant.a.; Puls.
TIMID: Bar.c.; Caust.
TONGUE, TRIANGULAR RED TIP: Rhus t.
TOUCHED, HATES TO BE: Kali c.
TREMBLING: Con.; Phos.
UNTIDY: Sul.
VIOLENT ATTACKS: Bell.
VOMITING: Lob.
WASHING, DISLIKE OF: Sul.
WATER, DISLIKE OF: Sul.
WEAK FEELING IN THROAT AFTER TALK-
   ING: Stann.
       "      "      "      " DURING TALKING:
   Stann.
WEAKNESS, MENTAL: Bar.c.
         "     PARALYTIC: Con.
WEEPS WHEN TELLING SYMPTOMS: Sep.
       "     "  THANKED: Lyc.
WEATHER, FEELS EVERY CHANGE: Nat.s.
WIND, EXCESSIVE ACCUMULATION IN
   LOWER ABDOMEN: Lyc.
     "  FEELS AS IF BLOWING ON SOME
   PART: Hep.s.
WORK, AVERSE TO: Sep.
WORRY: ars.a.
YELLOW SADDLE ACROSS NOSE: Sep.
YIELDING: Sil.

# MODALITIES

**Worse**

AIR, COLD: Ars.a.; Calc.c.; Caust.; Sep.
   " OPEN: Calc.c.; Carb.v.
APPLICATIONS, COLD: Ars.a.
   " WARM: Lyc.; Puls.
   " WET: Amm.c.
BATHING: Calc.c.
COFFEE: Kali c.
COLD: Carb.v.; Lob.
   " DRINKS: Ars.a.
   " TAKING: Con.
COLD, DAMP DWELLINGS: Nat.s.
DAMP: Sep.; Sil.
DRAUGHTS: Hep.s.
EATING, AFTER: Bar.c.; Bry.
EXERCISE, PHYSICAL or MENTAL: Con.
EXERTION: Con.; Phos.
FAINT ON SITTING UP: Bry.
HOT BED: Lyc.
JAR: Bell.
LIFTING: Rhus t.
LIMBS, LETTING HANG DOWN: Calc.c.
LOOKING DIRECTLY AT AN OBJECT: Cina.
LYING DOWN: Ant.t.; Bell.; Con.; Ipec.; Rhus t.
   " ON AFFECTED SIDE: Acon.; Bar.c.;
   Kali c.; Phos.
   " ON LEFT SIDE: Brom.; Kali c.; Nat.s.

LYING DOWN ON RIGHT SIDE: Stann.
MENSES, BEFORE: Con.
   " DURING: Con.
MOON, FULL: Calc.c.
   " NEW: Calc.c.
MOTION: Ferr.p.; Lob.
MOVE, ON BEGINNING TO: Rhus t.
MOVEMENT, SLIGHTEST: Bry.; Lob.
MUSIC: Acon.; Ambr.; Nat.s.
NOISE: Bell.
OVER-DRINKING: Nux v.
OVER-EATING: Nux v.
PERIODICALLY: Ipec.
PRESSURE OF CLOTHES: Calc.c
QUIET, WHEN: Iod.
REST, DURING: Samb.
SIDES, LEFT: Sep.
   " RIGHT: Ferr.p.; Iod.; Lyc.
SITTING: Rhus t.
   " IN WARM ROOM: Brom.
SLEEP: Samb.
STOOPING: Calc.c.
STRANGERS, IN PRESENCE OF CANNOT
    PASS STOOL OR URINE: Ambr.
STRAINING: Rhus t.
SOUP: Kali c.
THINKING OF SYMPTOMS: Bar.c.
TIME, MORNING: Ambr.; Amm.m.; Bry.;
   Calc.c.; Kali b.; Nux v.; Sil.; Sul.
   " NOON, AFTER: Bell.
   " AFTERNOON (ABDOMINAL
        SYMPTOMS): Amm.m.
   " 4–8 p.m.: Lyc.
   " EVENING: Amm.c.; Ant.t.; Carb.v.; Phos.
   " EVENING UNTIL MIDNIGHT: Brom.
   " NIGHT: Ars.a., Carb.v.; Cina; Ferr.p.
   " MIDNIGHT: Acon.

TIME, AFTER MIDNIGHT: Calc.c.
" 1–3 a.m.: Ars.
" 3 a.m.: Kali c.
" 3–4 a.m.: Amm.c.
" 4–6 a.m.: Ferr.p.
TOBACCO SMOKE: Acon.; Lob.
TOUCH: Bell.; Bry.; Ferr.p.
TWILIGHT: Phos.
UNCOVERING: Sil.
UNDRESSING: Kali b.
USING VOICE: Stann.
WALKING: Calc.c.
WARM DRINK: Phos.; Stann.
" FOOD: Phos.
" ROOM: Acon.; Ambr.; Iod.; Lyc.; Puls.
WARMTH: Ant.t.; Bry.
" OF BED: Sul.
WASHING: Amm.c.; Bar.c.
WEATHER, CHANGE OF: Phos.
" COLD: Lob.; Rhus.t.
" " WET: Calc.c.
" DAMP: Nat.s.
" " COLD: Ant.t.
" HOT: Bry.; Kali b.; Lyc.; Puls.
" MOIST: Sep.
" NIGHT AIR: Nat.s.
" SULTRY: Sep.
" SUMMER: Cina.
" TEMPERATURE, CHANGES, SUDDEN:
        Sticta p.
" WARM, DAMP: Brom.; Carb.v.
" WET: Amm.c.; Ars.a.; Rhus t.
" " GETTING, IN HEAT: Rhus t.
" " " WHEN SWEATING: Rhus t.
" WINDS, COLD, DRY: Acon.; Caust.;
        Hep.s.; Nux v.; Spong.
" " EAST: Sep.

WEATHER, MOIST, WARM: Ipec.
WORKING IN WATER: Calc.c.
WORMS: Cina.

# MODALITIES

**Better – Ameliorated by**
AIR DRY: Rhus t.
   " OPEN: Acon.; Amm.m.; Bar.c.; Iod.; Ipec.;
  Phos.
BENDING HEAD BACKWARDS: Sen.
BREAKFAST, AFTER: Calc.c.
COLD: Carb.v.
   " DRINKS: Ambr.
   " THINGS: Bry.
CONSTIPATED, WHEN: Calc.c.
COOL, BEING: Lyc.
COUGHING: Stann.
DARK, IN THE: Calc.c.; Con.
EATING, AFTER: Hep.s.
ERUCTATIONS: Carb.v.
EVENING: Lob.; Nux v.
EXERCISE: Brom.; Sep.
EXPECTORATING: Ant.t.; Stann.
FANNED, BEING: Carb.v.
FASTING: Con.
HEAT: Kali b.
LIMBS, DRAWING UP: Calc.c.
   " HANGING DOWN: Con.
LYING ON BACK: Calc.c.
LYING ON PAINFUL SIDE: Ambr.; Amm.c.;
  Bry.
   "    " STOMACH: Amm.c.

MIDNIGHT, AFTER: Lyc.

MOTION: Brom.; Con.; Kali c.; Lyc.; Rhus.t.; Samb.

" SLOW, IN OPEN AIR: Ambr.

NAP, AFTER: Nux v.

POSITION, CHANGING: Nat.s.

PRESSURE: Bry.; Con.; Nat.s.; Sep.; Stann.

REST: Bry.

RUBBING, FROM: Calc.c.

SEA, AT: Brom.

SEMI-ERECT: Bell.

SITTING ERECT: Ant.t.

" UP IN BED: Samb.

SWEATING: Sen.

WALKING ABOUT: Iod.

" SLOWLY IN OPEN AIR: Puls.

WARM FOOD: Lyc.

" DRINKS: Lyc.

WARMTH: Ars.a.; Hep.s.; Lob.; Sil.

WEATHER, DRY: Amm.c.; Nat.s.; Rhus t.

" " WARM: Calc.c.; Sul.

" HUMID: Sil.

" WARM, MOIST: Kali c.

" " WET: Nux v.

" WET: Sil.

WASHING, COLD: Lob.

WIND, BRINGING UP: Ant.t.

WRAPPING UP HEAD: Hep.s.; Sil.

# ASTHMA

Acon.; Ambr.; Ant.t.; Carb.v.; Con.; Cup.;
    Hep.s.; Kali c.; Lob.; Lyc.; Nat.s.; Nux v.;
    Rhus t.; Sep.; Sil.
ATTACKS, AFTER MIDNIGHT: Ars.a.; Ferr.p.
       "   AFTER SUPPRESSION OF ANY
            RASH OR MENSES: Puls.
       "   ALTERNATE WITH SKIN ERUP-
            TIONS: Sul.
       "   FROM EVERY DISORDERED
            STOMACH: Nux v.
       "   "   COMING ASHORE (SAILORS):
            Brom.
      " AT SEASIDE: Nat.s.
      " SINCE WHOOPING COUGH: Carb.v.
      " SUFFOCATING: Acon.; Ferr.p.
      " VIOLENT: Nat.s.; Spong.
      " WHEN TALKING: Dros.
      " WITH ANXIETY: Acon.; Ipec.
      "   " BRONCHIAL CATARRH: Nat.s.
      "   " COLLAPSE: Carb.v.
      "   " CONSTRICTION OF CHEST: Cup.
      "   " DISTENTION: Lyc.
      "   " EVERY CHANGE OF WEATHER:
            Carb.v.
      "   " FLATULENT DISTENSION: Carb.v.
      "   " HYSTERIA: Puls.

ATTACKS WITH WEAKNESS IN PIT OF
   STOMACH: Lob.
EVERY COLD ENDS IN: Sul.
BETTER, DAMP WEATHER: Hep.s.
     " SITTING UPRIGHT: Ars.a.
     " TALKING: Ferr.p.
     " WALKING SLOWLY: Ferr.p.
WORSE, AIR, DRY, COLD: Hep.s.
     " AFTER EATING: Nux v.
     " MORNING: Nux v.
     " NIGHT: Carb.v.
     " SHORTEST EXPOSURE TO COLD:
        Lob.
     " WALKING ABOUT: Ars.a.
     " WARM, DAMP WEATHER: Carb.v.

# BRONCHITIS

Acon.; Ant.t.; Bell.; Ferr.p.; Hep.s.; Lyc.; Phos.;
   Rhus t.; Sul.
IN INFANTS: Ipec.
IN OLD PEOPLE: Ant.t.; Ipec.; Rhus t.; Sen.;
   Ver.a.

# CHEST

BRONCHIAL CATARRH: Sen.
      "         " WITH WHEEZING: Spong.
CONSTRICTED, FEELS: Ars.a.; Brom.; Lyc.
DRYNESS IN, SENSATION OF: Acon.
HEAVINESS, FEELING OF: Sul.
ITCHING IN LEFT SIDE OF: Nat.s.
OPPRESSION OF: Ambr.; Amm.c.; Amm.m.;
   Dros.; Ferr.p.; Phos.; Rhus t.; Samb.
PAINS: BURNING: Amm.c.; Ars.a.; Brom.;
            Calc.c.; Carb.v.
  "    CRAMPING: Brom.
  "    SHOOTING: Acon.
  "    SORE: Amm.c.; Calc.c.; Ferr.p.; Nux v.;
            Puls.; Stann.
  "    STABBING: Ars.a.
  "    STICKING: Rhus t.
  "    STITCHING: Acon.; Bar.c.; Bell.; Bry.;
            Phos.; Sil.
  "    TINGLING: Con.
PRESSURE IN: Puls.
RATTLING WITH MUCUS: Carb.v.; Ipec.; Lyc.;
   Sen.
SENSIITIVE TO TOUCH: Calc.c.
TICKLING IN: Con.
TIGHT FEELING: Acon.; Calc.c.; Caust.; Ipec.;
   Phos.

TIRED FEELING: Amm.c.
WEAK FEELING: Ant.t.; Spong.; Stann.
WEIGHT, SENSATION OF: Sen.

# COUGH

ASTHMATIC: Amm.c.; Bar.c.; Brom.; Kali c.;
  Sep.; Spong.
BARKING: Ambr.; Amm.c.; Bell.; Spong.;
  Verat.a.
    " WITH GAGGING: Bry.
    "   " VOMITING: Bry.
CHOKING: Acon.; Dros.; Puls.; Samb.
CONTINUOUS: Amm.c.
CONVULSIVE: Acon.
CROUP: Acon.; Brom.; Ferr.p.; Hep.s.; Iod.;
  Kali b.; Samb.; Spong.
DEEP: Dros.; Lyc.
DRY: Acon.; Amm.c.; Ars.a.; Bar.c.; Bell.;
  Brom.; Bry.; Calc.c.; Caust.; Cina; Dros.;
  Ferr.p.; Hep.s.; Iod.; Ipec.; Kali c.; Nux v.;
  Phos.; Puls.; Rhus t.; Rum.; Sil.; Spong.;
  Stann.; Sticta p.
FULL OF MUCUS: Bar.c.; Caust.
GAGGING: Bry.; Carb.v.; Cina; Iod.; Ipec.; Kali
  c.; Puls.
HACKING: Acon.; Amm.m.; Ars.a.; Bry.; Con.;
  Kali b.; Nux v.; Sep.; Sen.
HARASSING: Dros.
HARD: Acon.; Bell.; Caust.; Ferr.p.; Kali c.;
  Phos.
HOARSE: Acon.; Cina; Dros.; Hep.s.
HOLLOW: Ambr.; Caust.; Cina; Lyc.

IRREPRESSIBLE: Spong.

IRRITATING: Acon.; Dros.

LOOSE: Amm.m.; Hep.s.; Nat.s.; Rhus t.; Samb.; Stann.; Sul.

LOUD: Spong.

NERVOUS: Ambr.

OBSTINATE: Sticta p.

PAROXYSMAL: Bry.; Carb.v.; Cina; Con.; Dros.; Rum.; Samb.

PERIODIC: Cina.

PERSISTENT: Calc.c.; Con.; Sil.

RACKING: Kali c.

RATTLING: Hep.s.

SCRAPING: Amm.m.

SHORT: Acon.; Ferr.p.

SPASMODIC: Ambr.; Bell.; Carb.v.; Cup.; Dros.; Ipec.; Nux v.; Rum.; Samb.

SUFFOCATIVE: Acon.; Bar.c.; Con.; Cup.; Iod.; Ipec.; Phos.; Puls.; Samb.; Sil.; Sul.

TEASING: Carb.v.; Ipec.; Nux v.; Puls.; Rhus t.; Rum.

TICKLING: Calc.c.; Dros.; Ferr.p.; Lyc.

TIGHT: Pros.; Rhus t.

WHEEZING: Ambr.; Ver.a.

WHOOPING: Ant.t.; Bell.; Brom.; Carb.v.; Cina; Con.; Cup.; Dros.; Ipec.; Nux v.; Sep.

WITH BURNING IN CHEST: Amm.c.

    "    BURSTING PAIN IN BACK: Sen.

    "    HEADACHE: Iod.; Lyc.; Nux v.

    "    HOARSENESS: Brom.

    "    INFLUENZA: Stann.

    "    NAUSEA: Ipec.

    "    PALPITATION: Amm.c.

    "    PROFUSE SALIVATION: Amm.m.

    "    RAWNESS OF CHEST: Caust.

    "    RETCHING: Iod.; Sep.

    "    SHORTNESS OF BREATH: Amm.c.

WITH SNEEZING: Kali c.
    "   SORENESS OF CHEST: Caust.
    "   STITCHING PAINS: Kali c.
    "   URINE ESCAPING: Puls.; Rum.; Ver.a.
    "   WORM SYMPTOMS:
VIOLENT: Spong.

# COUGH

**Aggravation – WORSE FROM:–**
AIR, COLD: Hep.s.; Phos.; Rum.; Spong.
    "   OPEN: Carb.v.
ATMOSPHERE DUSTY: Bell.
    "   CHANGING (temperature): Phos.
BREATH, A DEEP: Bell., Lyc.
CRYING: Bell.
DRAUGHTS: Kali c.
DRINKING: Kali c.
    "   COLD WATER: Bry.; Caust.; Cup.
EATING: Acon.; Bry.
    "   AFTER: Carb.v.
EMOTIONAL UPSET: Acon.
HILL, GOING DOWN: Lyc.
INDOORS: Iod.
INSPIRING: Brom.; Sticta.p.
LAUGHING: Bry.; Phos.
LYING DOWN: Acon.; Con.; Kali c.; Nat.s.;
    Puls.; Rum.; Sticta p.
        "     ON BACK: Amm.m.
        "     HEAD LOW: Spong.
        "     LEFT SIDE: Phos.
        "     RIGHT SIDE: Amm.m.
MOTION: Bry.; Kali c.
ODOURS, STRONG: Phos.
SLEEP, DURING: Acon.
SWALLOWING, EMPTY: Lyc.

TALKING: Acon.; Bell.; Bry.; Carb.v.; Phos.;
  Rum.; Sul.
TOBACCO SMOKE: Acon.; Bry.
UNCOVERING, ANY PART OF BODY: Hep.s.
WAKING: Ambr.
WALKING: Hep.s.
WARM ROOM, ON ENTERING: Bry.; Puls.;
  Ver.a.
WARMTH OF BED: Caust.
WEATHER, EVERY CHANGE IN: Bar.c.
    "      DAMP: Nat.s.
    "      WINDS, COLD: Hep.s.


## Amelioration – BETTER FROM:–

SITTING FORWARD: Kali c.
    "      UPRIGHT: Kali c.
WARM DRINKS: Nux v.; Sil.; Spong.
    "      FOOD: Spong.


## TIME AGGRAVATION

DAYTIME: Puls.
MORNING: Ambr.; Caust.; Sul.
EVENING: Carb.v.; Caust.; Sticta.p.
NIGHT: Bry.; Calc.c.; Dros.; Ferr.p.; Puls.;
  Sticta.p.; Sul.
    "  ON LYING DOWN: Bell.
BEDTIME UNTIL MIDNIGHT: Sep.
MIDNIGHT, AROUND: Ars.a.; Nux v.; Samb.
11 a.m.: Sul.
2–4 a.m.: Kali c.
3–4 a.m.: Nat.s.
3 a.m.: Amm.c.; Con.

# EXPECTORATION

BITTER: Puls.
BLAND: Puls.
BLOOD, CLEAR: Ferr.p.
BLOODY: Lyc.; Nux v.; Phos.; Sil.
COPIOUS: Nat.s.
FROTHY: Ars.a.; Sul.
GLUTINOUS: Kali b.
GRAY: Lyc.
GREENISH: Nat.s.; Puls.; Stann.; Sul.
LOOSE: Puls.
PROFUSE: Amm.c.; Kali b.; Sen.; Sep.; Spong.
PURULENT: Kali c.; Lyc.; Nat.s.; Phos.; Sil.;
    Sul.
RAISED WITH DIFFICULTY: Hep.s.
RUST COLOURED: Phos., Rhus.t.
SALTY: Lyc.; Phos.; Rhus t.
SCANTY: Acon.; Con.; Kali c.
SLIPS BACK WHEN SWALLOWED: Caust.
SOUR: Calc.c; Phos.
STICKY: Kali b.
STRINGY: Kali b.
SWEETISH: Stann.; Sul.
TASTES GREASY: Caust.
TENACIOUS: Kali b.; Kali c.; Rum.; Samb.;
    Sep.
THICK: Carb.v.; Lyc.; Puls.; Sep.; Sil.
THIN: Rum.

TOUGH: Rum.
WHITE: Sul.
WATERY: Rum.
YELLOW: Calc.c.; Dros.; Kali b.; Phos.; Sep.;
  Sil.
YELLOW/GREEN: Carb.v.

**Expectorate**
INABILITY TO: Lyc.; Sen

# RESPIRATION — BREATHING

ANXIOUS: Hep.s.

BREATHING FEELS AS IF THROUGH A
   SPONGE: Spong.

BREATHLESS: Ambr.; Ars.a.; Lyc.

BUBBLING: Ant.t.

CHOKING WHEN HAWKING MUCUS: Ambr.

DEEP BREATH, WANTS TO TAKE: Nat.s.

DIFFICULT: Acon.; Ambr.; Brom.; Bry.; Lob.;
   Spong.; Sul.

DIFFICULTY GETTING AIR INTO LUNGS:
   Brom.

GASPING: Samb.

INSPIRING DIFFICULT: Iod.

   "      RATTLING: Vera a.

   "      WHEEZING: Iod.

MOIST: Hep.s.

OPPRESSED: Acon.; Carb.v.; Sep.; Stann.

PAINFUL: Brom.

PANTING: Ferr.p.; Ipec.; Lyc.; Spong.

RAPID: Bry.; Iod.

RATTLING: Brom.; Calc.c.; Lyc.; Nat.s.

SHORTNESS OF BREATH: Acon.; Ambr.;
            Ant.t.; Con.; Cup.; Ferr.p.; Iod.;
            Ipec.; Nat.s.; Phos.; Samb.; Spong.;
            Stann.; Sul.

SHORTNESS OF BREATH WITH NAUSEA:
　　　　　　　　　　Lob.

"　　　　　" WITH VOMITING: Lob.
"　　　　　" WORSE RAPID
　　　　　　　　　MOTION: Sep.
"　　　　　" AFTER SLEEP: Sep.
"　　　　　" WALKING: Con.
"　　　　　"　　" AGAINST WIND:
　　　　　　　　Phos.

WHEEZING: Ant.t.; Ars.a.; Brom.; Carb.v.;
　　　　　　　　Hep.s.; Ipec.; Kali c.;
　　　　　　　　Lyc.; Spong.

WHISTLING: Spong.

# ADDITIONAL HINTS

'Feed a cold and starve a fever' is something I could never understand until I read an article which explained that the original saying was 'If you feed a cold you will have to starve a fever'. That makes sense!

When chest colds and wheezes are prevalent there is often a lot of catarrhal mucus. At this stage a day or two drinking plenty of fluid with very little (if anything) to eat, can bring about good improvement especially in children. Clearing the system in this way helps the remedies to work more quickly.

A call for something to eat usually marks an improvement.

Dairy products should be omitted as they are mucus forming. Instead diluted fruit juices or herb teas should be substituted. Vecon or Marmite with hot water are two enjoyable savoury drinks.

Starchy foods should be replaced with salads and vegetables; sweets, puddings and pastries with fresh fruit.

The body needs rest and relaxation when attacked by an illness in order that energy may be diverted to the healing process.